Reshaping your metabolism:

No diet,work on your mindset,loose the weight forever

By

Carrie Martin

Copyright © 2023

Table of content

INTRODUCTION

How does digestion influence your well-being?
Digestion is a term that depicts every one of the
synthetic responses in your body that keep your
body alive and working.
Your digestion is likewise answerable for
changing over supplements from the food
varieties you eat into fuel. This furnishes your
body with the energy it necessities to inhale,
move, digest food, course blood, and fix
harmed tissues and cells.
In any case, "digestion" is frequently used to
portray your basal metabolic rate or the number
of calories you copy very still.
The more your metabolic rate increases, the
higher you consume calories . Many elements
can influence your digestion, including your
age, diet, sex, body size, and well-being status
(1Trusted Source).
There are a few proof-based techniques that
can assist with expanding your digestion to help

weight the executives and generally speaking wellbeing.

These are some methods for expanding your digestion.

1. Eat a lot of protein at each dinner

Eating food can briefly expand your digestion for a couple of hours.

Eating more protein can help you so you burn more calories. It can likewise assist with giving you a more prominent feeling of totality and forestall indulging.

2. Hydrate

Water can assist you with shedding pounds and keeping them off. It briefly expands your digestion and helps top you off before dinners

3. Do an extreme focus exercise

Stirring up your work-out daily schedule and including a couple of focused energy exercises can support your digestion and assist you with consuming fat

4. Lift weighty things

Lifting loads can help fabricate and hold muscle while diminishing muscle versus fat. Higher amount of muscle will bring about a better chance to burn fat

5. Stand up more

Sitting for quite a while consumes not many calories and may adversely influence your well-being. Have a go at standing up or going for strolls consistently or putting resources into a standing work area

6. Drink green tea or oolong tea

Drinking green tea or oolong tea might expand your digestion. These teas may likewise assist you with getting thinner and keeping it off, assuming that is your objective, however, research is blended.

7. Eat zesty food sources

Eating zesty food could be useful for supporting your digestion and assisting you with keeping a moderate weight. In any case, the digestion-supporting impact of fiery food sources is minuscule

8. Get a decent night's rest

Absence of rest can diminish the number of calories you consume, alter the manner in which you process sugar, and disturb your hunger-managing chemicals

9. Drink coffee

Drinking espresso can altogether build your digestion and may assist you with shedding pounds assuming that is your objective.

How much time it takes to accelerate your
digestion can change in view of various
variables, including your:
diet
movement level
wellbeing status
While a portion of the tips recorded above
might assist with expanding your digestion
rapidly, others might take more time.
Furthermore, these systems ought not to be
viewed as a handy solution, yet rather, they
ought to be integrated into an arrangement with
well-being advancing advantages that
incorporate eating a supplement thick eating
regimen joined with active work and ideal rest
to accomplish enduring outcomes.

CHAPTER 1
MUSCLE IS MONEY

In the event that you can support a lifting program and eat a calorie deficiency, your body will actually want to pull from its fat stores to both fuel itself and possibly fabricate bulk. Focusing on food sources wealthy in protein is a vital part of both losing muscle versus fat and building muscle simultaneously.

There are various motivations behind why somebody might set out on another exercise program. A couple of the most widely recognized wellness objectives are to shed pounds and fabricate muscle; on the off chance that you wish to do both, you are possibly seeking after-body recomposition.

The subtleties and construction of your exercise plan will generally be directed by your essential wellness objective. For instance, in the event that your objective is a fat misfortune, your attention will be on consuming calories and controlling your caloric admission to make the energy deficiency important to consume fat. Then again, assuming you want to beef up and assemble bulk, you will need to participate in strength-preparing exercises that help hypertrophy (expansions in muscle size) and up your supplement admission to help muscle development.

What is body recomposition?
Expanding your lean weight and diminishing your muscle versus fat are both body recomposition objectives. Body arrangement alludes to the general level of fat tissue (fat) and fit weight (muscle, bone, organs, nerves, blood, connective tissues, and so on) you have. Body recomposition includes changing your body piece, as a rule via losing muscle-to-fat ratio and building muscle (slender weight).

Could you at any point add muscle while consuming fat?
To lose muscle versus fat, you must be in a calorie deficiency, and that implies that you're consuming fewer calories than you're consuming consistently. It takes a deficiency of

3,500 calories to lose one pound of put-away muscle-to-fat ratio. In the event that you ponder this throughout the span of seven days, this likens to losing one pound of fat assuming you consume 500 additional calories each day than you're eating

To advance muscle development, likewise called hypertrophy, your muscles need both a boost as well as an important asset. The "improvement" for muscle development for the most part drops via strength preparation (lifting loads) with an exercise program of moderate over-burden.

Weighty opposition preparation makes minuscule harm to your muscle strands, basically making small tears in the muscle tissue. This harm animates the body to start the muscle reparative cycle. This interaction is called myofibrillar protein union, yet you'll likewise at times hear it called muscle protein blend.

Here is where the "vital assets" part of muscle development becomes possibly the most important factor.

The course of the muscle protein blend requires satisfactory protein and energy (calories). Proteins from the food sources you eat are separated into their structure blocks, called amino acids. These amino acids are moved to the muscle tissue after your exercise and collected into new reparative proteins.

How could I eat to acquire muscle and lose fat?

Proof proposes that the best eating routine for building muscle in a calorie deficiency is to consume 2.3-3.1 g/kg of lean weight each day of protein, 15%-30% of your complete calories from fat, and the rest of your calories from sugars. It's ideal to separate these supplements into three to six feasts each day. The dinner just previously and just after your obstruction preparing exercise ought to contain 0.4-0.5 g/kg of body weight of protein. For instance, in the event that you weigh 75 kg (165 pounds), you ought to consume at least 75 X 2.3g = 173g of protein each day and around 75 x 0.5 = 37.5g just after your exercise.

Once more, remember that your pace of fat misfortune will be slower assuming you're attempting to assemble muscle simultaneously. Research shows a rate that doesn't surpass 0.7% of muscle versus fat each week.

CHAPTER 2
TRAIN YOUR BRAIN.

Ways You Can Prepare Your Mind to lose weight.

1. Ditch the scale fixation.

No, truly. At the point when you're fixated on the scale, the number you see could mean the contrast between an incredible day and a total breakdown, which sets you up for deplorable outcomes.

However, you'll need to gauge progress and make your weigh-ins sensible. In the event that you normally step on the scale one time each day, consider changing to week after week or every other month weigh-ins.
In particular, don't allow the scale to control you. It's simply a number, and it's not generally intelligent of your actual advancement and difficult work.

2. Shift your belief.

All through your lifetime, you've likely heard a few unique convictions about food. Your folks might have urged you to clean your plate, in any event, when you were full. You might have watched your mom or father moan about being on a careful nutritional plan. Or on the other hand, perhaps you've heard your companions say that they "shouldn't" eat either or that they "ought to" go to the rec center.

These assertions can have an enormous effect on how you view weight reduction.

Record all the judgment-based proclamations you can imagine and toss out any that are causing you to continue to feel regretful or awful about yourself. Your endeavors to get healthier ought to be a positive space, not loaded up with self-hatred or incalculable guidelines to observe

The world is suffocating in data on well-being, sustenance, and exercise. From liver purging to lentils, leotards to lycra, low cal to lavage, and piece size to paleo, new weight reduction patterns are springing up quicker than you can sauté kale. However, 95% of individuals who attempt to get in shape placed everything back on, in addition to more, in something like a year

of beginning any kind of weight reduction
system. Why?
Since the vital figure is effective weight, the
board has been neglected: the cerebrum.

The mind is our control community. All aspects
of the body adhere to the signs and guidelines
conveyed by the mind. The mind decides why,
how, and where muscle versus fat is put away.
The mind drives our digestion, hunger, food
decisions, inspiration to work out (or not), and
chemical creation. So set aside your feast plan
and begin with the accompanying Psyche Plan.

- Rather than zeroing in on the thing you
  ought to eat, direct your concentration
  toward why you are eating. No less than
  30% of our eating is eager for non-eating.
  We eat in light of the fact that we're
  miserable, furious, exhausted, desolate,
  pushed, discouraged, hesitating,
  celebrating, sympathizing, and
  pondering, the rundown is unending. On
  the off chance that you eat when you're
  not eager, your body needn't bother with
  the energy and will store it as an

abundance muscle to fat ratio. Thusly before you go after food, ask yourself 'Am I truly ravenous or am I attempting to change how I'm feeling?' Assuming you're really eager, eat. Assuming that it's a personal explanation, read stage two.

- One of the most engaging and mending things we can do instead of solace eating, is to just sit with our feelings without smothering them or occupying ourselves from them. Indeed, it's awkward. Be that as it may, distress doesn't hurt us. It's simply awkward. We could do without feeling awkward, yet the distress doesn't stand the test of time. In the event that you can sit discreetly and let yourself feel the upsetting inclination for only a couple of moments, you'll be flabbergasted at how it disseminates and you really feel empowered by the cycle. Furthermore, you'll never again feel like the sugar hit or anything that it was you were going to eat.

- . Allow yourself to sit idle. One of the most well-known triggers for eagerness for non-eating is expecting to enjoy some time off based on the thing you're doing. We feel regretful for halting in light of the fact that we live in a general public that causes us to feel we must be useful constantly. So we search for reasons and food is a simple decision. You don't have to eat to legitimize having a break.

- At the point when you eat, simply eat. Try not to do anything more in light of the fact that the cerebrum can zero in on each thing in turn and you'll miss the signs from your body about whether the food really concurs with you and the amount of it you really want. Focus on the smell, surface, and nuances of flavor. You'll partake in your food all the more however wind up eating less in light of the fact that you're fulfilled sooner. The more we taste, the less we want. The blows individuals away. A great many people believe that the more they partake in their food, the more they will eat. The inverse is valid. The mystery is to relish each significant piece.

- . Figure out how to eat until you're 80% full. The Japanese call this 'hara hachi bu'. The explanation is that it requires around 20 minutes for the many signs from your stomach and fat cells to arrive in your mind and let you know that you've had enough. So assuming you eat until you're 80% full, quickly you'll find you're really 100% full and you'll be happy you halted when you did.

- Get a normal decent night's rest. Lack of sleep drives up every one of the chemicals that increment appetite and sugar desires. Also expecting to set yourself up with food since you're worn out.

CHAPTER 3
MANAGE YOUR BLOOD SUGAR

How Balancing out Glucose Assumes a Major Part in Weight Reduction

It is authoritatively mid-spring in Northern Nevada, and that implies individuals are getting out into the daylight and making arrangements for the mid-year season. For some, this incorporates shedding the quarantine layers of sweat and perhaps a couple of additional pounds. As a chiropractic practice that spotlights health and generally speaking well-being, we get gotten some information about weight reduction. One of the greatest contributing variables to weight reduction is glucose. This is frequently ignored in light of the fact that individuals take a gander at calories and fat while attempting to manage down, however, sugar is one of the greatest boundaries to individuals hitting their objective weight.

What is glucose?

Your blood glucose level is the proportion of convergence of glucose present in the blood.

The body gets glucose from the food we eat and is the principal wellspring of energy in the body. The ingestion, stockpiling, and creation of glucose are directed continually by complex cycles including the small digestive tract, liver, and pancreas.

The pancreas produces insulin, delivering it after an individual consumes protein or carbs. The insulin sends an abundance of glucose to the liver as glycogen. The pancreas likewise delivers a chemical called glucagon, which does something contrary to insulin, raising glucose levels when required. At the point when the body needs more sugar in the blood, the glucagon flags the liver to transform the glycogen back into glucose and delivery it into the circulation system.
At the point when your eating routine is in balance, these frameworks work in the show. The issue happens when the body needs insulin, has it excessively, or on the grounds that the body isn't working actually. Cells might foster resistance to insulin, making it vital for the pancreas to create and deliver more insulin to bring down your glucose levels. In the long

run, the body can neglect to create sufficient insulin to stay aware of the sugar coming into the body.

How truly does high glucose forestall weight reduction?

Weight reduction happens when we exhaust more energy than we consume (calories). Yet, it additionally happens when we have adjusted glucose and no overabundance of insulin. The overabundance of insulin is made because of a lot of sugar in our bodies, and this insulin flood lets our bodies know that a lot of energy is accessible and that they ought to quit consuming fat and begin putting away it. By controlling your levels and keeping them within sound reach (between 80 mg/ml and 120 mg/ml), you will handle carbs and proteins for energy as opposed to having them put away as fat.

Instructions to test your glucose levels

You ought to counsel a clinical expert in the event that you suspect your levels might be out of equilibrium. They can suggest either an expert or at-home test for you to quantify your glucose level.

Food varieties that assist with balancing out your glucose levels
The least complex method for balancing out your glucose levels is to be aware of what you eat. Sugar conceals in a ton of our food, particularly in the event that it is handled. At the point when you center around eating entire food sources (things that are basically developed starting from the earliest stage), will have a lot better glucose level. It is likewise essential to eat on a normal timetable and not skip feasts so you don't experience a glucose crash and reach for a handled nibble to pick you back up.

WHOLE FRUITS
Specifically consuming blueberries, grapes, and apples can help essentially bring down your gamble of creating Type 2 diabetes, a recent report found. Except for melons and pineapples, most natural products have low glycemic record (GI) scores and are a decent decision while balancing out glucose levels.

YAMS AND SWEET POTATOES

Yams can assist with settling or lower glucose levels and they are without a doubt an invigorating, nutritious food with a low GI score. Individuals can substitute yams or sweet potatoes for potatoes in various dishes, from fries to meals.

WHOLE WHEAT OR PUMPERNICKEL BREAD

Truth be told bread. While most bread ought to be kept away from while balancing out glucose in view of the sugars, entire wheat, and pumpernickel have lower GI scores since they go through less handling, leaving them with more fiber that eases back assimilation and assists with settling glucose levels.

OATS

Oats are a superfood. They decrease glucose and insulin reactions after dinners, further, develop insulin responsiveness, keep up with glycemic control, and diminish fats in the blood.

NUTS

Most nuts make a healthful and low GI nibble ideal for assisting you with feeling full, giving you energy, and not spiking glucose. Nuts additionally contain elevated degrees of plant proteins, unsaturated fats, and different supplements like cancer prevention agents and potassium.

Vegetables

Beans, chickpeas, peas, and lentils are vegetables that incorporate fiber, protein, and complex sugars to give you energy, encourage you longer, and even lower the gamble of coronary illness. Be careful to eat your vegetables entirety. For instance, make a pot of beans at home as opposed to opening a can. Those canned and handled beans can contain hills of stowed-away sugar that will most likely upset your glucose levels.

 Understanding your body's course of putting away sugar and paying attention to your body's requirements will support by and large well-being and ideal capability. While your general calorie admission is significant when you are hoping to get in shape, watching your sugar utilization can get you improved results, quicker. What's more, you will make a better body generally.

CHAPTER 4
SLEEP IS YOUR MAGIC PILL

How much rest you get might be similarly as significant for weight reduction as your eating regimen and exercise. Proof shows that rest might be the missing variable for some individuals attempting to get thinner.

Sadly, many individuals aren't getting sufficient rest.

As a matter of fact, around 35% of US grown-ups are dozing less than 7 hours most evenings, as per the Habitats for Infectious Prevention and Counteraction (CDC). Not sleeping up to 7hours in the evening is not enough.

Two Different Ways Rest Might Assist You With Getting Fit

- May assist you with keeping away from weight gain related to short rest

Short rest — typically characterized as less than 6-7 hours — has been over and over-connected to a higher weight file (BMI) and weight gain.

One investigation of 20 examinations including 300,000 individuals found a 41% expanded stoutness risk among grown-ups who dozed less than 7 hours in the evening. Conversely, rest was not a figure for the improvement of corpulence in grown-ups who dozed longer (7-9 hours in the evening).

One more review viewed short rest term as fundamentally connected with a more prominent midsection periphery, which is a sign of the gathering of stomach fat

Different investigations have tracked down comparable outcomes

Studies have additionally tracked down comparable relationships between youngsters and teenagers.

In a new survey of 33 observational and mediation studies, a short rest span was related to an expanded gamble of weight. Curiously, for each extra hour of rest, BMI scores diminished

One more survey of numerous observational examinations found short rest term was related to an essentially higher gamble of corpulence in these different age gatherings

Outset: 40% expanded risk
Youth: 57% expanded risk
Center adolescence: 123% expanded risk
Immaturity: 30% expanded risk
One significant audit found that short rest
length improved the probability of corpulence in
youngsters by 30-45%
However the absence of rest is just a single
figure for the improvement of stoutness,
research recommends it adversely influences
hunger levels, impacting an individual to eat
additional calories from high-fat and high-sugar
food varieties.
It might do this by influencing hunger chemical
levels, expanding ghrelin, which causes you to
feel hungry, and diminishing leptin, which
encourages you
Ghrelin is a chemical delivered in the stomach
that signs hunger in the mind. Levels are high
before you eat, which is the point at which the
stomach is vacant, and low after you eat. Leptin
is a chemical let out of fat cells.

- May help moderate your appetite

Getting enough sleep may help prevent
increases in calorie intake and appetite that can
happen when you're sleep deprived.
It is discovered that people who doesn't have
enough sleep report having a large appetite
and a lots of calories consumed daily
In fact, one discovery found that those who
doesn't get enough sleep consumed an
additional 385 calories per day, where most of it
are fat
Another discovery showed that not getting
enough sleep leads to high increases in
hunger, food cravings, portion sizes,and fat
intake..
When you do not get quality sleep, the body
makes less leptin and more ghrelin, leaving you
hungry and increasing your appetite.

CONCLUSION

At this point, you will have an action plan for forward movement. You might decide to dive into the deep end by Simultaneously Incorporating changes to the type of foods you eat, how you exercise and move Your body your sleep schedule, and Your mental health practices. Or you might decide to start Simple with something you Can Sustain such as meal-prepping lunches for work Instead of relying on take-outs. Either way, you will be ready to learn the art of losing weight by reprogramming Your mind for a change.